KICKING SUGAR TO THE CURB

A PROVEN 7-STEP PROCESS TO END DIETING

BY 

CHITARO LINCOLN

Table of Contents

Introduction 4

Chapter One...6

   The Dangers of Sugar....................................6

Chapter Two 10

   Understanding Dieting 10

Chapter Three 14

   Step 1 - Creating a Support System 14

Chapter Four...18

   Step 2 - Identifying Triggers 18

Chapter Five 22

   Step 3 - Setting Realistic Goals.................22

Chapter Six 26

   Step 4 - Finding Healthy Alternatives.........26

Chapter Seven 30

   Step 5 - Managing Stress............................30

Chapter Eight..34

Step 6 - Developing a Positive Mindset......................34

Here are some tips to help you develop a positive

mindset. 34

Chapter Nine 38

Step 7 - Celebrating Success 38

Here are some tips to help you celebrate success: ...38

Introduction

Here will explore the harmful effects of sugar on our bodies and how it leads to unhealthy dieting habits. We will provide a proven 7-step process to help you kick sugar to the curb and put an end to unhealthy dieting practices.

In this book, we have provided a comprehensive 7-step process to help you kick sugar to the curb and end unhealthy dieting habits. We hope that by following these steps, you will be able to establish a healthy relationship with food and live a healthier, happier life. Remember, this process is a journey, and it takes time, patience, and persistence to achieve success. Good luck!

Chapter One

The Dangers of Sugar

This chapter provides an overview of the negative effects of sugar on our health. It explores the relationship between sugar and chronic diseases such as obesity, diabetes, and heart disease. It also examines how sugar affects our blood sugar levels, insulin production, and energy levels. This chapter provides an important foundation for understanding the harmful effects of sugar and why it is important to kick the sugar habit.

Sugar is a type of carbohydrate that is found naturally in many foods such as fruits, vegetables, and dairy products. However, the sugar that is most concerning for our health is added sugar - the sugar that is added to processed foods and drinks during manufacturing, cooking, or preparation.

There are several dangers associated with consuming too much added sugar. One of the most significant risks is the development of obesity. When we consume sugary foods and drinks, our bodies convert the sugar into glucose, which raises our blood sugar levels. This increase in blood sugar triggers the release of insulin, a hormone that helps the body store glucose as fat. If we consume too much added sugar, our bodies may end up storing excess glucose as fat, leading to weight gain and obesity over time.

Furthermore, consuming excessive amounts of added sugar can also lead to type 2 diabetes. When we eat sugar, our blood sugar levels spike, causing our bodies to release insulin to regulate blood sugar levels. Over time, the constant need for insulin can lead to insulin resistance, where the body becomes less responsive to insulin. As a result, the body produces even more insulin to try to control blood sugar levels, which can eventually lead to type 2 diabetes.

Sugar has also been linked to heart disease, one of the leading causes of death worldwide. Consuming too much added sugar can raise triglyceride levels in the blood, which is a type of fat that is associated with an increased risk of heart disease. In addition, a high sugar diet can lead to inflammation in the body, which has also been linked to an increased risk of heart disease.

Other dangers of sugar include dental decay, mood swings, and increased risk of certain types of cancer. Consuming too much sugar can cause dental decay and cavities, as sugar provides a food source for bacteria that can damage tooth enamel. High sugar diets can also cause mood swings and irritability, as the spikes and crashes in blood sugar levels can affect our mood and energy levels. Finally, some studies suggest that consuming high amounts of sugar may increase the risk of certain types of cancer, such as pancreatic and colon cancer.

Overall, the dangers of sugar are significant and far-reaching. While it's important to remember that sugar is not inherently bad, and it is okay to enjoy sugary treats in moderation, it's important to be mindful of the amount of added sugar in our diets and to make healthy choices that prioritize whole, nutrient-dense foods.

Chapter Two

Understanding Dieting

This chapter explores the different types of diets and why they often fail. It examines how dieting can lead to unhealthy habits such as binge eating and restrictive eating patterns. It also discusses the importance of establishing a healthy relationship with food. This chapter helps readers understand why dieting isn't the solution to a healthy lifestyle, and why it's important to focus on creating a healthy relationship with food.

Dieting is the practice of controlling one's food intake to achieve a desired outcome, such as weight loss, improved health, or athletic performance. While there are many different approaches to dieting, all diets involve some degree of calorie restriction or manipulation of macronutrient intake (carbohydrates, protein, and fat).

One of the most common types of diets is a low-carbohydrate diet, which restricts the intake of carbohydrates and increases the intake of protein and fat. Low-carb diets are often used for weight loss, as they can lead to a reduction in appetite and overall calorie intake. However, they can also be effective for managing certain medical conditions such as diabetes and epilepsy.

Another popular type of diet is the Mediterranean diet, which is characterized by a high intake of fruits, vegetables, whole grains, and healthy fats such as olive oil and nuts. The Mediterranean diet has been associated with a reduced risk of heart disease, stroke, and other chronic diseases.

There are also many fad diets that promise quick weight loss or other health benefits but may not be sustainable or effective in the long term. For example, the ketogenic diet, which involves very low carbohydrate intake and high fat intake, has gained popularity in recent years for its weight loss and other health benefits, but it can be difficult to maintain in the long term and may have negative side effects such as nutrient deficiencies.

It's important to note that dieting can also have negative effects on mental and emotional health. Restrictive diets can lead to feelings of deprivation, anxiety, and guilt around food, which can contribute to disordered eating patterns such as binge eating or orthorexia (an obsession with "clean" or "healthy" eating).

Overall, while dieting can be effective for achieving certain health or performance goals, it's important to approach it with caution and to prioritize balanced, sustainable eating habits. A registered dietitian or other qualified healthcare professional can provide personalized guidance and support for individuals looking to make dietary changes.

Chapter Three

Step 1 - Creating a Support System

This chapter explores the importance of having a support system when trying to kick sugar and end dieting. It provides strategies for building a support system, including seeking support from friends and family, joining support groups, and seeking professional help. This chapter helps readers understand the importance of having support and accountability when making lifestyle changes.

When embarking on a journey to kick sugar to the curb and end dieting, one of the most important steps is to create a support system. A support system can consist of friends, family members, healthcare professionals, or anyone else who can provide encouragement and accountability on your journey.

Having a support system can be especially helpful when facing challenges or setbacks, such as cravings for sugary foods or feelings of discouragement. Your support system can offer words of encouragement, provide helpful tips and advice, or simply be a listening ear when you need to vent.

To create a support system, start by identifying people in your life who you trust and feel comfortable confiding in. This may include friends or family members who are also interested in healthy living, a registered dietitian or other healthcare professional, or a support group focused on overcoming sugar addiction or disordered eating.

Once you've identified potential members of your support system, reach out to them, and let them know about your goals and how they can help you. This may involve asking for specific types of support, such as going for a walk together instead of meeting for coffee or checking in with you regularly to see how you're doing.

It's also important to communicate openly and honestly with your support system about any challenges or struggles you may be facing. This can help to prevent feelings of shame or guilt and can create a safe and supportive environment for you to share your experiences and receive feedback and guidance.

In addition to creating a support system of people, it can also be helpful to seek out resources such as books, online communities, or apps that provide information and support for your goals. These resources can supplement your personal support system and provide additional guidance and inspiration.

Overall, creating a support system is a critical step in kicking sugar to the curb and ending dieting. By surrounding yourself with people who understand your goals and can provide encouragement and accountability, you can stay motivated and focused on your journey towards a healthier, happier life.

Chapter Four

Step 2 - Identifying Triggers

This chapter explores the different triggers that lead to sugar cravings and unhealthy eating habits. It provides strategies for identifying these triggers and developing strategies to avoid them. This chapter helps readers understand the importance of being aware of their triggers and how to manage them.

Step 2 in the process of kicking sugar to the curb and ending dieting is identifying triggers. Triggers are the situations, emotions, or circumstances that make you more likely to crave sugar or engage in unhealthy eating behaviors.

Common triggers include stress, boredom, social situations, and certain foods or smells that are associated with sugary treats. For example, if you always reach for a candy bar when you're feeling stressed at work, stress can be a trigger for your sugar cravings.

Identifying your triggers is an important step because it allows you to anticipate situations that may lead to unhealthy behaviors and develop strategies to cope with them. Here are some steps to help you identify your triggers:

Keep a food diary: Write down everything you eat and drink, as well as the time of day, your mood, and any other relevant information. This can help you identify patterns and associations between your food choices and your emotions.

Notice when you crave sugar: Pay attention to when you feel the strongest cravings for sugar. Is it always at a certain time of day or in response to a particular emotion or situation?

Consider your environment: Think about the places and situations where you are most likely to crave sugar. Is it at home, at work, or when you're out with friends?

Reflect on past experiences: Consider times when you've struggled with sugar cravings in the past. What was going on in your life at the time? What helped you overcome the cravings?

Once you've identified your triggers, you can start to develop strategies to cope with them. For example, if stress is a trigger for your sugar cravings, you might try practicing relaxation techniques such as deep breathing or meditation. If boredom is a trigger, you might try finding new hobbies or activities to keep yourself busy.

It's important to remember that identifying your triggers is an ongoing process, and it may take time and practice to develop effective coping strategies. Be patient and compassionate with yourself as you work towards a healthier relationship with food and sugar.

Chapter Five

Step 3 - Setting Realistic Goals

This chapter explores the importance of setting realistic goals when trying to kick sugar and end dieting. It provides an overview of the SMART goal-setting framework and how it can be applied to this process. This chapter helps readers set achievable goals and track their progress.

Step 3 in the process of kicking sugar to the curb and ending dieting is setting realistic goals. Having clear and achievable goals can help keep you motivated and focused on your journey towards a healthier lifestyle.

When setting goals, it's important to make them specific, measurable, achievable, relevant, and time bound. Here are some tips to help you set realistic goals:

Be specific: Instead of setting a general goal like "I want to eat less sugar," be specific about what you want to achieve. For example, "I want to limit my daily sugar intake to 25 grams."

Make them measurable: Set goals that you can track and measure over time. For example, you might track your daily sugar intake using a food diary or app.

Keep them achievable: Make sure your goals are realistic and achievable for your current lifestyle and circumstances. Setting unrealistic goals can lead to feelings of failure and discouragement.

Ensure they are relevant: Your goals should be relevant to your overall health and wellness. Consider how achieving your goals will benefit your physical and mental health.

Set a deadline: Give yourself a specific deadline for achieving your goals. This will help you stay motivated and focused on making progress.

When setting goals, it's also important to celebrate your successes along the way. Recognize and acknowledge your achievements, no matter how small they may seem.

This can help you stay motivated and continue making progress towards your larger goals.

It's also important to remember that setbacks and challenges are a natural part of the journey towards a healthier lifestyle. If you encounter obstacles or struggle to meet your goals, be gentle with yourself and use it as an opportunity to learn and grow.

In summary, setting realistic goals is an important step in kicking sugar to the curb and ending dieting. By making your goals specific, measurable, achievable, relevant, and time-bound, you can stay motivated and focused on your journey towards a healthier, happier life.

Chapter Six

Step 4 - Finding Healthy Alternatives

This chapter explores healthy alternatives to sugar and processed foods. It provides examples of nutrient-dense whole foods and healthy snack and meal options. This chapter helps readers understand the importance of nourishing their bodies with healthy foods and provides practical ideas for healthy eating.

Step 4 in the process of kicking sugar to the curb and ending dieting is finding healthy alternatives. One of the challenges of cutting out sugar is finding alternative foods and drinks that satisfy your cravings while also being healthy.

Here are some tips to help you find healthy alternatives to sugar:

Focus on whole foods: Incorporate whole foods into your diet, such as fruits, vegetables, lean proteins, and whole grains. These foods are nutrient-dense and can help satisfy your hunger and cravings without relying on sugar.

Use natural sweeteners: Replace processed sugar with natural sweeteners such as honey, maple syrup, or stevia. These options are lower in calories and can be used in moderation to satisfy your sweet tooth.

Experiment with flavors: Try experimenting with different flavors and spices to add variety to your meals. For example, cinnamon can add a natural sweetness to your food, while spices such as cumin or paprika can add depth and complexity to your dishes.

Drink water: Stay hydrated by drinking plenty of water throughout the day. Water can help keep you feeling full and satisfied, and it's a healthier alternative to sugary drinks.

Read labels: Pay attention to food labels and look for products that are low in added sugars. Some packaged foods, such as cereals and granola bars, can be high in added sugars, so it's important to read the labels and choose healthier options.

Find healthy snacks: Snacks can be a challenging area when cutting out sugar, but there are plenty of healthy options available. Try snacking on nuts, seeds, fresh fruits, or vegetables with hummus or other healthy dips.

Finding healthy alternatives to sugar may take some trial and error, but it's an important step in developing a healthier relationship with food. Be patient with yourself and experiment with different foods and flavors to find what works best for you.

In summary, finding healthy alternatives to sugar is an important step in kicking sugar to the curb and ending dieting. By focusing on whole foods, using natural sweeteners, experimenting with flavors, drinking water, reading labels, and finding healthy snacks, you can satisfy your cravings while also nourishing your body with healthy, nutrient-dense foods.

Chapter Seven

Step 5 - Managing Stress

This chapter explores the relationship between stress and unhealthy eating habits. It provides strategies for managing stress, including mindfulness practices, exercise, and self-care activities. This chapter helps readers understand the importance of managing stress for overall health and wellbeing.

Step 5 in the process of kicking sugar to the curb and ending dieting is managing stress. Stress can have a significant impact on your eating habits and overall health, so it's important to find ways to manage stress in a healthy way.

Here are some tips to help you manage stress:

Identify your stress triggers: Take note of situations or events that tend to cause stress for you. Once you identify your stress triggers, you can work on avoiding or managing them in a healthy way.

Practice relaxation techniques: Relaxation techniques such as deep breathing, yoga, or meditation can help reduce stress and promote feelings of calm and relaxation.

Exercise regularly: Exercise is a great way to reduce stress and improve your overall health. Even a small amount of physical activity each day can help lower stress levels.

Get enough sleep: Lack of sleep can increase stress levels and lead to poor eating habits. Make sure you're getting enough rest each night to help manage stress and maintain a healthy lifestyle.

Seek support: Talking to friends, family, or a therapist can help reduce stress and provide a supportive environment to help you achieve your goals.

Prioritize self-care: Taking time for yourself to relax and engage in self-care activities can help reduce stress and improve your overall wellbeing.

By managing stress in a healthy way, you can improve your overall health and reduce the likelihood of turning to sugary foods or other unhealthy habits to cope with stress.

In summary, managing stress is an important step in kicking sugar to the curb and ending dieting. By identifying your stress triggers, practicing relaxation techniques, exercising regularly, getting enough sleep, seeking support, and prioritizing self-care, you can reduce stress levels and maintain a healthy lifestyle.

Chapter Eight

Step 6 - Developing a Positive Mindset

This chapter explores the importance of developing a positive mindset when trying to kick sugar and end dieting. It provides an overview of the role of self-talk and how to shift negative thought patterns to positive ones. This chapter helps readers understand the importance of mindset for achieving long-term lifestyle changes.

Step 6 in the process of kicking sugar to the curb and ending dieting is developing a positive mindset. The way we think about ourselves and our ability to make positive changes in our lives can have a significant impact on our success.

Here are some tips to help you develop a positive mindset.

Practice positive self-talk: Replace negative self-talk with positive affirmations. Instead of telling yourself you can't do something, tell yourself that you can and will achieve your goals.

Focus on progress, not perfection: Instead of striving for perfection, focus on making progress towards your goals. Celebrate small victories and use them as motivation to keep going.

Surround yourself with positivity: Surround yourself with people and things that make you feel positive and uplifted. This can include positive affirmations, supportive friends and family, and uplifting music or books.

Set realistic expectations: Setting realistic expectations for yourself can help prevent feelings of disappointment or failure. Don't set unrealistic goals that are impossible to achieve, instead, set achievable goals that will help you make progress towards your overall goal.

Visualize success: Visualize yourself achieving your goals and imagine how it will feel to reach your desired outcome. This can help keep you motivated and focused on your goals.

Practice gratitude: Focusing on what you're grateful for can help shift your mindset towards positivity and help you stay motivated and focused on your goals.

By developing a positive mindset, you can overcome self-doubt and negative self-talk, and stay motivated towards your goals. This can help you make positive changes in your life, including cutting out sugar and ending dieting.

In summary, developing a positive mindset is an important step in kicking sugar to the curb and ending dieting. By practicing positive self-talk, focusing on progress, surrounding yourself with positivity, setting realistic expectations, visualizing success, and practicing gratitude, you can develop a positive mindset and achieve your goals.

Chapter Nine

Step 7 - Celebrating Success

This chapter explores the importance of celebrating success when trying to kick sugar and end dieting. It provides examples of ways to celebrate success and the benefits of positive reinforcement. This chapter helps readers stay motivated and encourages them to recognize and celebrate their achievements.

Step 7 in the process of kicking sugar to the curb and ending dieting is celebrating success. Celebrating your successes, no matter how small, is an important part of the process and can help keep you motivated and focused on your goals.

Here are some tips to help you celebrate success

Acknowledge your progress: Take time to reflect on the progress you've made towards your goals. This can include weight loss, improved energy levels, or simply making healthier food choices.

Reward yourself: Treat yourself to a non-food reward when you reach a milestone or achieve a goal. This can include buying yourself a new outfit, taking a relaxing bath, or treating yourself to a massage.

Share your success: Share your success with others, whether it's friends and family, a support group, or on social media. Celebrating with others can help keep you motivated and accountable.

Set new goals: Once you've achieved one goal, set a new one. This will help you continue making progress and prevent you from falling back into old habits.

Stay positive: Celebrating success is important, but it's also important to stay positive when faced with setbacks. Remember that setbacks are a natural part of the process and focus on getting back on track.

By celebrating your successes, you can stay motivated and focused on your goals, and continue making positive changes in your life.

In summary, celebrating success is an important step in kicking sugar to the curb and ending dieting. By acknowledging your progress, rewarding yourself, sharing your success, setting new goals, and staying positive, you can celebrate your successes and stay motivated towards achieving your overall goal of ending dieting and living a healthier lifestyle.